Contents

INTRODUCTION

Nothing will make you a more valued and accomplished colorist than the ability to perform corrective work. To err is human, but to correct is divine.

Corrective Hair Coloring: A Hands-On Approach will help you achieve a high level of professionalism in corrective color through both color theory and hands-on experiments that allow you to learn by experiencing. In this text, the discussion is limited to permanent hair color, where corrective situations most commonly arise.

Current market research shows that before the end of the twentieth century, 40 percent of total salon revenues will come from hair color. While there are no statistics available on hair color revenues lost through mistakes, if just 5 percent of your clients are dissatisfied, it could be financially devastating. On the other hand, each time you are able to correct another's hair coloring mistakes, statistics do show that you'll gain a loyal client for life, which translates into financial success.

The majority of professional cosmetologists are currently working with color methodology that was developed between 1930 and 1950. But the chemicals in hair color and what is known about them have undergone many complex changes. As technology advances, it becomes even more imperative that the cosmetologist advance with it and stay attuned to new developments.

The purpose of this book is to provide an overview of all those developments and the current education necessary to become an expert corrective hair colorist, regardless of the hair color product you choose to use. As you progress through color theory, selection of base colors, overviews of lighteners and bleaches, and selection of hydrogen peroxide volumes, you'll increase your hair color confidence. By working through the experiments, you'll develop and expand the analytical skills that will allow you to approach any situation in the salon with self-assurance.

Once you've completed the book, you'll want to keep it as a reference manual for daily use. The chemical selection charts included can be used with any manufacturer's products to achieve beautiful results.

Corrective coloring is nothing to be intimidated by, nor need it be confusing. By following the guidelines in this book, advanced color services will become one of your strong points and, with that expertise, your future success as a colorist is ensured.

1 Basic Color Theory

Learning Objectives

After completing this chapter, you should be able to:

- define primary, secondary, and tertiary colors.
- explain how molecular weight of colors affects hair color.
- demonstrate how new colors are created.
- explain how to neutralize unwanted color.
- list colors according to the order they are found in the cuticle.
- identify the color components of any end color result.

The understanding of basic color theory is essential to analyze a client's color or perform a color correction.

Primary colors are basic, or true, colors. The primary colors are, in the order of their atomic weights, blue, red, and yellow. (See Color Plate 1.) Understanding the order and size is essential to understanding hair color theory. The order and size of the primary colors reflect the laws of physics. To illustrate this, observe what happens during the lift cycle when going from black (level 1) to light blond (level 9).

Blue is the only cool primary, and when it is added to any primary, secondary, or tertiary color it is dominant. The resulting new color will also be cool. (See Color Plate 2.) Its molecular size or pigment weight is very important; it is the primary color with the largest molecular size and the heaviest pigment weight. Because of this, blue is closest to the cuticle layer and is easiest to remove. The blue primary color dissipates, leaving the hair shaft first because of its location on the hair shaft. When the hair is oxidized by ammonia in a perm or hair-coloring solution, the hair shaft expands sufficiently to allow the blue molecule to oxidize and escape.

The next primary color is red, and, again, its molecular size and placement within the cortex of the hair shaft is important. It explains why red is difficult to remove during lightening. Red is positioned deeper in the hair shaft than blue, so in order to remove it, you must swell or expand the hair shaft large enough and for a long enough time to allow oxidation to affect the red molecule, so it will dissipate into the atmosphere.

Last, but by no means least, of the primaries is yellow, which is found deepest within the hair shaft. The yellow molecule is very hard to remove completely for the same reasons that red is. To completely remove yellow, bleach is the surest — and in most cases the easiest — way to complete removal.

When all three primary colors are present in equal proportions, the result is neutral brown or neutral blond, depending on the amount of the pigment present. (See Color Plate 3.)

Secondary colors are created when any two primaries are mixed together in equal parts. (See Color Plate 4.) If you add the opposite of any secondary color, you neutralize it, and it becomes a neutral brown or neutral blond, again depending on the amount of pigment present in the hair shaft.

Tertiary colors are created by combining a primary color with a secondary color located on either side of it on the color wheel, in equal proportions. (See Color Plate 5.)

The following explains how to neutralize any unwanted color in the spectrum. (See Color Plate 6.)

Locate on the color wheel the color opposite of the one you wish to neutralize. Then add an equal amount of that color pigment, and you will achieve a neutral color. This color will be brown or blond, again depending on the depth of pigment it contains.

For example:

- Blue Violet + Yellow Orange = Neutral Brown
  or Neutral Blond

- Blue Violet + Yellow Orange = Neutral Brown
  or Neutral Blond

- Blue Violet + Yellow Orange = Neutral Brown
  or Neutral Blond

To enhance any color in the spectrum, add any other color you have chosen in equal proportions. (Remember that certain color combinations are undesirable in hair color.)

Understanding these basic theories is critical to performing corrective hair coloring. If any concept is not clear to you, go back and review it before continuing further.

Remember, any color you use, whether in a bottle or tube, contains dye molecules of primary, secondary, or tertiary colors. Simply match these base colors with the shade you wish to achieve for the desired results. See the Base Color Test in Chapter 2 for a method of determining base colors.

Experiment Instruction Sheets

Creating Secondary Colors

Objective

To observe and document the results of mixing the three primary colors to obtain secondary colors.

Primary Watercolors Needed
- Blue
- Red
- Yellow

Materials Needed
- Three bowls
- One large piece of construction paper
- Paint brush
- Bowl of water
- Towel

Procedure

1. Measure ¼ teaspoon of blue watercolor and ¼ teaspoon of red watercolor into a mixing container.

2. Once these colors have been combined, use the paint brush to mix thoroughly and apply some of this mixture to the construction paper.

3. Mix ¼ teaspoon of blue watercolor and ¼ teaspoon of yellow watercolor.

4. Once these colors have been combined, use the paint brush to mix thoroughly, and apply some of this mixture to the construction paper.

5. Mix ¼ teaspoon of red watercolor and ¼ teaspoon of yellow watercolor.

6. Once these colors have been combined, use the paint brush to mix thoroughly and apply some of this mixture to the construction paper.

7. Mount and label the results of each test on the Experiment Results Sheet at the end of the chapter.

8. Answer Review Questions for this experiment at the end of the chapter.

Experiment Instruction Sheets

Creating Tertiary Colors

Objective

To combine the primary colors and secondary colors to create tertiary colors.

Primary and Secondary Colors

- Blue
- Red
- Yellow
- Violet
- Green
- Orange

Materials Needed

- Three bowls
- One large piece of construction paper
- Paint brush
- Bowl of water
- Towel

Procedure

1. Mix ¼ teaspoon of blue watercolor and ¼ teaspoon of violet watercolor.

2. Once these colors have been combined, use the paint brush to mix thoroughly, and apply some of this mixture to the construction paper.

3. Mix ¼ teaspoon of red watercolor and ¼ teaspoon of orange watercolor.

4. Once these colors have been combined, use the paint brush to mix thoroughly, and apply some of this mixture to the construction paper.

5. Mix ¼ teaspoon of yellow watercolor and ¼ teaspoon of green watercolor.

6. Once these colors have been combined, use the paint brush to mix thoroughly, and apply some of this mixture to the construction paper.

7. Mix ¼ teaspoon of blue watercolor and ¼ teaspoon of green watercolor.

8. Once these colors have been combined, use the brush to mix thoroughly, and apply some of this mixture to the construction paper.

9. Mix ¼ teaspoon of red watercolor and ¼ teaspoon of violet watercolor.

10. Once these colors have been combined, use the paint brush to mix thoroughly, and apply some of this mixture to the construction paper.

11. Mix ¼ teaspoon of red watercolor and ¼ teaspoon of orange watercolor.

12. Once these colors have been combined, use the paint brush to mix thoroughly, and apply some of this mixture to the construction paper.

13. Mix ¼ teaspoon of yellow watercolor and ¼ teaspoon of orange watercolor.

14. Once these colors have been combined, use the brush to mix thoroughly, and apply some of this mixture to the construction paper.

15. Mix ¼ teaspoon of red watercolor and ¼ teaspoon of violet watercolor.

16. Once these colors have been combined, use the paint brush to mix thoroughly, and apply some of this mixture to the construction paper.

17. Mount and label the results of each test on the Experiment Results Sheet at the end of the chapter.

18. Answer Review Questions for this experiment at the end of the chapter.

Experiment Results Sheets and Review Questions

Creating Secondary Colors

Experiment Results Sheet

Blue and Red

Blue and Yellow

Red and Yellow

Blue and Red —
Color Achieved: _____

Blue and Yellow —
Color Achieved: _____

Red and Yellow —
Color Achieved: _____

Experiment Results Sheets and Review Questions

Creating Secondary Colors

Review Questions

1. What are the three primary colors?

2. Why are they called primaries?

3. What are secondary colors, and how are they created?

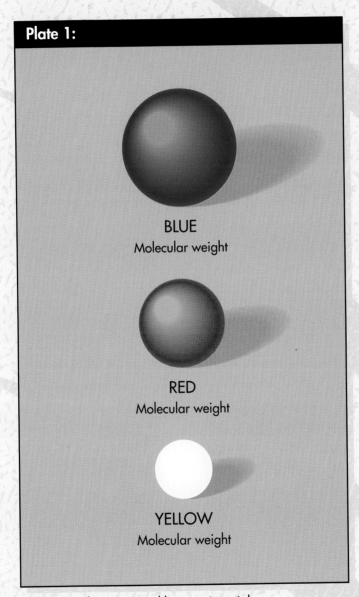

Primary colors arranged by atomic weight.

Plate 2:

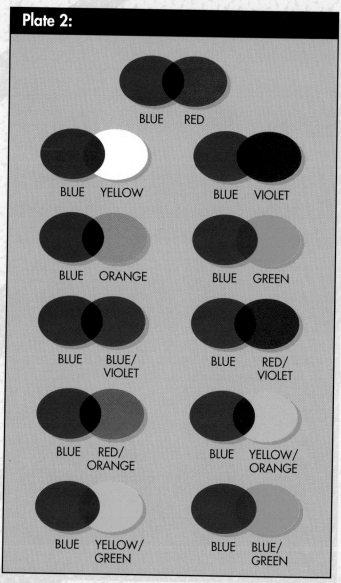

BLUE   RED

BLUE   YELLOW

BLUE   VIOLET

BLUE   ORANGE

BLUE   GREEN

BLUE   BLUE/
VIOLET

BLUE   RED/
VIOLET

BLUE   RED/
ORANGE

BLUE   YELLOW/
ORANGE

BLUE   YELLOW/
GREEN

BLUE   BLUE/
GREEN

Blue shown in combination with any secondary or
tertiary color creates a cool result.

Plates 3 & 4:

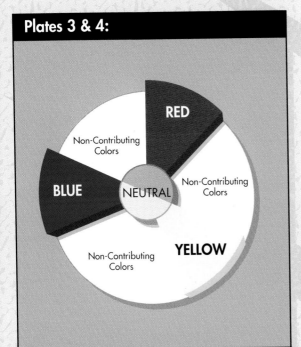

Red, blue and yellow, combined equally create neutral.

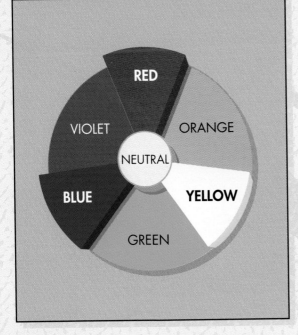

Secondary colors are created from equal parts of two primaries.

Plates 5 & 6:

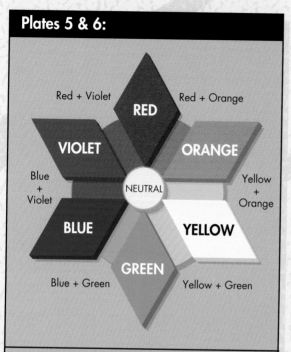

Wheel showing how the combination of primary and secondary colors create tertiary colors.

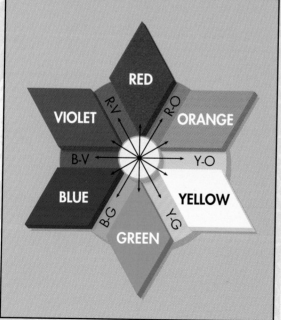

Complete color wheel with arrows to indicate which colors neutralize others.

4. How do primaries and secondaries relate to hair color?

5. List the primary colors in order of molecular weight.

6. Describe ways in which the color wheel is used by hair colorists.

Experiment Results Sheets and Review Questions

Creating Tertiary Colors

Experiment Results Sheet

Blue and Violet

Red and Orange

Yellow and Green

Blue and Green

Red and Violet

Red and Orange

Yellow and Orange

Red and Violet

List the cool tertiary colors:

List the warm tertiary colors:

List the neutral tertiary colors:

Experiment Results Sheets and Review Questions

Creating Tertiary Colors

Review Questions

1. Which tertiary colors are not appropriate for use in hair color, or not pleasing to the eye?

2. How do you neutralize blue/green?

3. How are tertiary colors positioned on the color wheel?

4. What is the role of depth of pigment?

5. What is present in all tertiary colors? In what proportions is it present?

2 The Level System

Learning Objectives

After completing this chapter, you should be able to:

- identify the base color of any hair color product.
- explain oxidation.
- identify shades of color within a base.
- select the correct level of color to achieve desired results.
- determine the level of virgin or chemically treated hair.
- explain remaining pigment and how it affects levels of color.
- solve color formulation problems.

This chapter will describe the level system, remaining pigment contribution, and shades of color. It will also explore determination of color formulation, which will be discussed at length in a later chapter. Understanding the use of hair color is essential before attempting hair color application.

The level system is a method of categorizing hair color numerically in relation to depth of color and lifting capabilities. Most hair color manufacturers use the level system as a way of standardizing hair color charts and numbering their color bottles and/or tubes. The level system ranks hair color from 1 to 10, level 1 being black or the darkest brown possible, and level 10 being the lightest blond possible before white. (See Fig 2.1.)

1 *Black Color*	**6** *Brown Color* Red Brown Gold Brown Ash Brown
2 *Brown Color* Warm Brown Ash Brown Natural Brown	**7** *Blond Color* Red Blond Gold Blond Ash Blond Natural Blond
3 *Brown Color* Warm Brown Ash Brown Natural Brown	**8** *Blond Color* Red Blond Gold Blond Ash Blond Natural Blond
4 *Brown Color* Red Brown Ash Brown Natural Brown	**9** *Blond Color* Red Blond Gold Blond Ash Blond Natural Blond
5 *Brown Color* Red Brown Gold Brown Ash Brown Natural Brown	**10** *Blond Color* Gold Blond Ash Blond Platinum Blond (Violet) Natural Blond

Figure 2.1.

The level system. The various shades are listed for the levels.

Some color companies, particularly those based in Europe, do use numbers higher than 10, but for the most part, levels above 10 have very little color pigment in them, minimizing or negating deposit. They generally react the same as a mild oil or cream bleach does.

Remaining Pigment Contribution

Primary, secondary, and tertiary colors can be found at any level of natural hair color. (See Fig. 2.2.) Remaining pigment contribution is the color that will be left in the hair after the lifting process. Knowing the colors that will be present at a given level of color ensures that you will select the proper base color formulation to either neutralize or enhance the desired color.

One of the problems you will face when coloring hair is that most color charts display color selections on white hair swatches. This falsely leads colorists to believe that the color shown is the color they will attain. The charts don't take into consideration the pigment contributed from the natural hair that will remain during the lifting cycle. (Note: Figure 2.2 is designed for use as a rule of thumb. New companies are introducing color lines at a staggering rate, making specific quitclaims subject to constant change.)

Oxidation

The percentage of lift in any color is directly related to its ammonia content.

The percentage of deposit is directly related to the dye content in the color bottle or tube.

The percentage of dye content in the bottle or tube is also known as pigment weight. The more dye molecules in the bottle, the more depositing capabilities the color has. The action of depositing dye or color molecules into the cortex of the hair shaft is partly triggered by oxidation, which is achieved by adding hydrogen peroxide (H_2O_2) to the color.

THE LEVEL SYSTEM

Dark Browns			Medium-Light Browns			Dark & Light Blonds			Light Blonds		
1	2	3	4	5	6	7	8	9	10	11	12
Remaining Pigment Contribution											
B L U E	B L U E	V I O L E T	R E D	R E D	R E D	O R A N G E	Y E L L O W	Y E L L O W	P A L E	P A L E	W H I T E
	V I O L E T		V I O L E T		O R A N G E		O R A N G E		Y E L L O W	E S T	
										Y E L L O W	
Primary Tertiary Colors			Primary Tertiary Colors			Secondary Tertiary Colors					
90% DEPOSIT 10% LIFT			50% DEPOSIT 50% LIFT			90% LIFT 10% DEPOSIT					
% LIFT=AMMONIA CONTENT % DEPOSIT = DYE CONTENT											
Volume of H_2O_2 used should be consistent with the time needed and the percent of lift designated by the manufacturer.											
1 volume of H_2O_2 = 1 minute of time											

Figure 2.2.

Remaining pigment contribution left in the hair during the lifting process for the various levels.

The dye molecule in any permanent color is too large to penetrate the cuticle of the hair shaft without first altering its structure with hydrogen peroxide. (See Fig. 2.3.) Since without hydrogen peroxide the dye will only stain the cuticle layer, understanding what happens when you add hydrogen peroxide to color is essential.

After the hydrogen peroxide is added to the color, it begins to oxidize, or lose an oxygen molecule. This creates heat in and on the hair shaft, which expands the cuticle layer so that the color or dye molecules can penetrate.

Once the hydrogen peroxide is completely oxidized, it turns into water (H_2O), and its chemical action stops. The color molecules return to their original structure and become part of the structure of the cortex. The cuticle closes, trapping the dye or color molecules inside. The color process is complete.

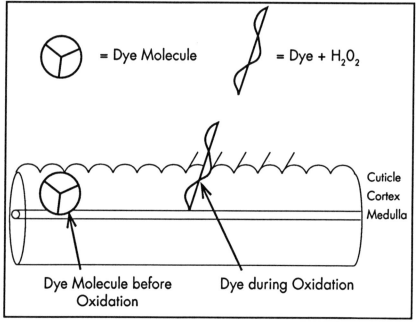

Figure 2.3.

Enlarged hair shaft with changed and unchanged dye molecules in cortex.

Natural Pigment Granules

Pigment granules are present in the cortex of natural hair. The specific pigments inside the granules are as follows:

Black...melanins

Brown ....melanins

Red ....oximelanins

Yellow.......................................oximelanins

Various combinations of these are present in all natural hair. Most importantly, these are combinations of the primary colors, as discussed in Chapter 1.

Shades of Color

The concept of shades of color causes much confusion and this confusion causes multiple problems. A shade of color is the specific tonal quality of any given color within the ten-level system. There can be as many as four shades within each level. Manufacturers decide how many shades will be within each level when they develop their color lines. Examples are ash, gold, red, or a neutral shade at any given level of color. Shades of color can be named whatever the manufacturer chooses to call them, but if you can determine the base color, you will not be confused by the different names given a shade within a level. Do not assume that the name given a color by the manufacturer indicates the base color. When in doubt, use the test on the following page to determine it.

Color Formulation

The previous pages covered vital concepts for performing basic color work. To determine color formulation and effectively color hair, begin by answering the following questions:

1. What level of color is the client's hair?
2. What level of color does the client desire?
3. What shade or color does the client prefer?

   (Examples: ash, gold, red, or neutral.)
4. What base color will neutralize or enhance the client's color choice?
5. Does the client have fine, medium, or coarse hair?
6. Has the client's hair been chemically treated?

Once these standard questions are answered, select a color with the proper base color, and that has the correct lifting and depositing capabilities to ensure success. In the event you don't know the base color of your product, use the following test to determine it.

Base Color Test

1. When using tube color, mix a small amount in a bowl and add an equal amount of 10 volume hydrogen peroxide.
2. Apply the mixture to a piece of cotton, and wait for 10 minutes.
3. At the end of this time, you will see the true color base.

1. When using liquid color, mix a small amount in a bowl and add an equal amount of 5 volume hydrogen peroxide.

2. Apply the mixture to a piece of cotton and wait 5 minutes.

3. At the end of this time, you will see the true color base.

Example 1

Consider the following example, for use when lifting in the level system:

Client's preferred color is a level 7.

Client's natural color is a level 4.

Subtract the natural color level from the level the client wishes to achieve.

Add the difference to the preferred color level. This will give you the proper color level to use to achieve the desired results:

Preferred level of color	Level 7 Blond
Natural level of color (subtract)	- Level 4 Brown
Difference	= 3 levels

Preferred level of color	Level 7 Blond
Difference (add)	+ 3 levels
Level to use	= Level 10 Blond

The level of color to be used is a level 10 blond with a blue base. The base color must be blue, or the orange (remaining pigment) will show through. (Refer to Fig. 2.2.)

Explanation

The client is a level 4 brown and wants to be a level 7 blond. The difference between the natural level of color (where the client is) and the desired level of color (where the client wants to be) is three levels. If you use a level 7 color, will you achieve the desired results?

No! You must use a color that will account for the difference between the client's natural level and the client's preferred level.

A level 10 color is the correct choice, with the appropriate base color. However, using a level 10, which contains only pale yellow dyes, will not keep the orange in a level 7 from showing through. (See Fig. 2.4.) The result will be brassiness.

What can you do to neutralize it? Add a color accent from the manufacturer or add a maximum of 1/4 oz. of weekly rinse in your color formula. One manufacturer has a preformed dye molecule that is added to its color product line for this purpose.

Example 2

Here is another example of lifting in the level system:

Client's preferred color is a level 9.

Client's natural color is a level 4.

Subtract the natural color level from the level the client wishes to achieve, and add the difference to the preferred color level. This will give you the proper color level to use for the desired results.

Level System
Remaining Pigment Chart

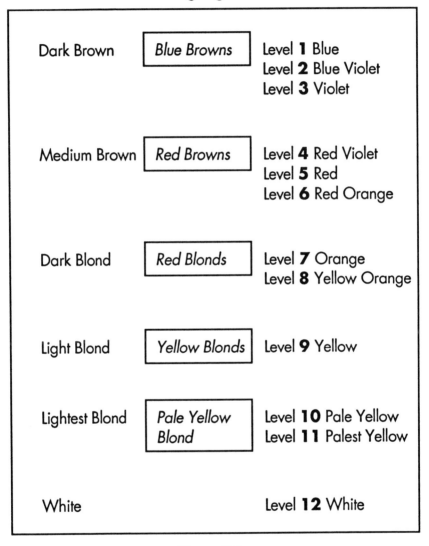

Figure 2.4.

When a client wishes to change levels, be aware of the pigment that shows through at the new level.

Preferred level of color	Level 9 Blond
Natural level of color (subtract)	<u>- Level 4 Brown</u>
Difference	= 5 Levels

Preferred level of color	Level 9 Blond
Difference (add)	<u>+ 5 Levels</u>
Level to use	= Level 14 Blond

Explanation

Example 2 demonstrates a common lift problem that can be addressed before applying color using a one-step color process.

The client is a level 4 and wishes to achieve a level 9. The difference between these levels is 5, which when added to level 9 equals 14 — a level that does not exist within the level system.

What will solve this dilemma? Use the highest level available in the color line you currently use, then add a maximum of 1/4 oz. oil or cream lightener to the formula. Since you will now need more time to process the color, use a higher volume of hydrogen peroxide to provide extra time. Remember, one minute of oxidation time equals one volume of hydrogen peroxide. (Refer to Fig. 2.2.)

Most manufacturers would recommend a two-step process; for this information see what your color company recommends.

However, any color results can be achieved by analytical thinking and reviewing the information in this book.

Experiment Instruction Sheets

Determining Natural Level
of Virgin Hair

Objective

To analyze natural hair within the context of the level system.

Hair Supplies Needed

2 samples of virgin, human hair in the following color levels:

- Brown
- Blonde

Labeling Hair Samples

Label each sample according to its natural level.

Materials Needed

- One color swatch chart

Procedure

1. Break up into teams of four. Use the Experiment Results Sheet at the end of the chapter, and lay a small section of hair from one team member on the paper to identify what level it is. (Choose a blond or brunette team member; arrive at a consensus.)

2. Use the color swatch ring to determine if your identification is correct.

3. Mount and label each of the results from blond or brunette team members on the Experiment Results Sheet at the end of the chapter.

4. Answer the end-of-chapter Review Questions for this experiment.

   Note: If it is difficult to find a large number of students who have virgin hair, rearrange team sizes accordingly but limit the tests within a group to four people, as this is the number the Experiment Result Sheet accommodates.

Experiment Instruction Sheets

Determining Level of Chemically Treated Hair

Objective

To determine the level of chemically-treated hair within the context of the level system.

Hair Samples Needed

2 samples of chemically treated human hair in the following color levels:

- Brown
- Blond

Labeling Hair Samples

Label each sample according to its level.

Materials Needed

- One color swatch ring

Selection and Results

1. Break the class into teams of four. Use the Experiment Results Sheet at the end of the chapter, and lay a small section of hair from one team member on the paper to identify what level it is. Choose a blond or brunette team member; arrive at a consensus.

2. Use the color swatch ring to determine if your identification is correct.

3. Label each of the results from all team members who have chemically treated, blond or brunette hair on the Experiment Results Sheet at the end of the chapter.

4. Answer the end-of-chapter Review Questions for this experiment.

Experiment Results Sheets and Review Questions

Determining Natural Level of Virgin Hair

Experiment Results Sheet

Subject 1 Level   Subject 2 Level

Subject 3 Level   Subject 4 Level

Number of Levels Displayed: _____

Experiment Results Sheets and Review Questions

Determining Natural Level of Virgin Hair

Review Questions

1. What is the level system, and how is it used in formulating color?

2. What is remaining pigment contribution?

3. Which pigments remain at level 6?

4. Why are color-chart hair swatches not indicative of true end results?

5. List the levels that natural brunettes could fall into.

6. Explain why a colorist must be aware of remaining pigment at any level.

Experiment Results Sheets and Review Questions

Determining Level of Chemically Treated Hair

Experiment Results Sheet

Subject 1 Level   Subject 2 Level

Subject 3 Level   Subject 4 Level

Number of Levels Displayed: _____

Experiment Results Sheets and Review Questions

Determining Level of Chemically Treated Hair

Review Questions

1. What is the difference between shade and level?

2. Give names to the levels you see in this experiment; include the base in your name.

3. What is melanin?

4. What determines lift? Deposit?

5. How does oxidation occur?

3 Hydrogen Peroxide and Its Uses

Learning Objectives

After completing this chapter, you should be able to:

- describe how hydrogen peroxide reacts with ammonia.
- explain what is meant by volume of peroxide.
- calculate the lifting or depositing capabilities of peroxide when mixed with any given amount of color or water.
- explain and demonstrate correct peroxide volume choices for a predetermined amount of lift or deposit.

Hydrogen peroxide plays an essential role in corrective coloring. This chapter includes a detailed explanation of types of hydrogen peroxide (H_2O_2) and their roles in the color process. It also includes charts for breaking down the numerous volumes of hydrogen peroxide.

Hydrogen peroxide, in its pure state, is a syrupy, clear liquid. This chemical is a violently active compound that is much too strong for ordinary use.

Cream hydrogen peroxides contain small amounts of acids, which lower the product's pH and helps stop decomposition. Hydrogen peroxide will oxidize if it isn't stabilized or will turn into water (H_2O).

Oxidation hair color dyes have a small amount of ammonia water in their bottles or tubes. This neutralizes the acid stabilizers in the hydrogen peroxide, so the product can release oxygen molecules. This is called oxidation.

Some colorists fear using volumes of hydrogen peroxide. The most important thing to understand is that *volume* means "by weight." Since volume is a measure of weight, anything that is added to any volume of hydrogen peroxide will change the weight. For example, if you add 1 oz. of water to 1 oz. of 20 volume hydrogen peroxide, you will have 2 oz. of 10 volume hydrogen peroxide. The reason for this is that they have like weights.

If you add 2 oz. of color to 2 oz. of 20 volume hydrogen peroxide, the weight of the 20 volume hydrogen peroxide decreases because of the added color. This is what occurs during color formulation.

The mathematical formula below can be used to determine whether you are using the proper volume of hydrogen peroxide for the purposes of the manufacturer.

$$\frac{2 \text{ oz. of hair color} + 2 \text{ oz. of } H_2O_2}{4 \text{ (total quantity)}}$$

then

$$\text{Divide } \frac{20 \text{ (volume of } H_2O_2)}{4 \text{ (total quantity)}} = 5 \text{ (lift or deposit capabilities)}$$

Remember, add the total quantity of product used, then divide that sum into the volume of hydrogen peroxide used. The result is the lift or depositing capabilities of the hydrogen peroxide that you are using in your color formula.

Uneven and Odd Volume Numbers

When using uneven or odd numbers, divide the number 4 into the volume of hydrogen peroxide that is used in your formula. The following common examples will simplify your math and give you the corrected volume of hydrogen peroxide you will use in most situations.

For:	1 oz. color	For:	1 oz. color
	1 oz. 20 vol.		1 oz. additive
	Use: 20/4 (5)		1 oz. 20 volume
			Use: 20/4 (5)
For:	1 ½ oz. color	For:	1 oz. color
	1 ½ oz. 10 vol.		1 oz. 30 vol.
Use:	10/4 (2.5)	Use:	30/4 (7.5)
For:	1 oz. color	For:	1 ½ oz. color
	1 oz. 40 vol.		1 ½ oz. 40 vol.
Use:	40/4 (10)	Use:	40/4 (10)

Remember, in the cases of uneven or odd numbers, you are not adding, but always dividing 4 into the volume of peroxide.

When diluting high volumes of hydrogen peroxide, use the following charts:

130 Volume Hydrogen Peroxide Dilution Chart

For 16 oz. Total Quantity

12 ½ oz. of H_2O_2 + 3 ½ oz. of H_2O (water) = 16 oz. of 100 volume H_2O_2

7 ½ oz. of H_2O_2 + 8 ½ oz. of H_2O (water) = 16 oz. of 60 volume H_2O_2

6 ½ oz. of H_2O_2 + 9 ½ oz. of H_2O (water) = 16 oz. of 50 volume H_2O_2

5 oz. of H_2O_2 + 11 oz. of H_2O (water) = 16 oz. of 40 volume H_2O_2

3 ½ oz. H_2O_2 + 12 ½ oz. of H_2O (water) = 16 oz. of 30 volume H_2O_2

2 ½ oz. H_2O_2 + 13 ½ oz. of H_2O (water) = 16 oz. of 20 volume H_2O_2

1 ¼ oz. H_2O_2 + 14 ¾ oz. of H_2O (water) = 16 oz. of 10 volume H_2O_2

100 Volume Hydrogen Peroxide Dilution Chart

For 10 oz. Total Quantity

6 oz. of H_2O_2 + 4 oz. of H_2O (water) = 10 oz. of 60 volume H_2O_2

5 oz. of H_2O_2 + 5 oz. of H_2O (water) = 10 oz. of 50 volume H_2O_2

4 oz. of H_2O_2 + 6 oz. of H_2O (water) = 10 oz. of 40 volume H_2O_2

3 oz. of H_2O_2 + 7 oz. of H_2O (water) = 10 oz. of 30 volume H_2O_2

2 oz. of H_2O_2 + 8 oz. of H_2O (water) = 10 oz. of 20 volume H_2O_2

1 oz. of H_2O_2 + 9 oz. of H_2O (water) = 10 oz. of 10 volume H_2O_2

Use this next chart to determine the deposit or lift required to achieve each level of color. Then, select the appropriate formula and note the mixtures that correspond to those formulas.

Level System

Hydrogen Peroxide Chart

Levels of Color

1 2 3	4 5 6	7 8 9	10 11 12
90% Deposit	50% Deposit	10% Deposit	
10% Lift	50% Lift	90% Lift	
2.5–6 volume H_2O_2	7–11 volume H_2O_2	12–18 volume H_2O_2	
Depositing Formula	Medium Lift Formula	High Lift Formula	
2 oz. color	2 oz. color	2 oz. color	
2 oz. 20 vol. H_2O_2	2 oz. 40 vol. H_2O_2	2 oz. 60 vol. H_2O_2	
4/20 = 5 vol.	4/40 = 10 vol.	4/60 = 15 vol.	
Depositing Formula	Medium Lift Formula	High Lift Formula	

Experiment Instruction Sheet

Varying Volumes of Hydrogen Peroxide

Objective

To observe and document the results after mixing variable volumes of hydrogen peroxide and water.

Materials Needed

- One beaker of water (distilled)
- One bottle of 100 volume H_2O_2
- One mixing bottle (8 oz. color bottle)
- One bottle of 40 volume H_2O_2

Procedure

Experiment #1: Selection and Formulation

Use the 8 oz. color bottle for mixing. Mix ½ oz. 100 volume hydrogen peroxide with 4 ½ oz. of distilled water.

1. Using the chart for 100 volume peroxide dilution, find the results of this experiment.

2. Label your results appropriately on the Experiment Results Sheet at the end of the chapter.

Procedure

Experiment #2: Selection and Formulation

Use the 8 oz. color bottle and mix 2 oz. of 100 volume H_2O_2 with 3 oz. distilled water.

1. Use the 100 volume hydrogen peroxide chart to find the appropriate results.

2. Label and document results on the Experiment Results Sheet at the end of the chapter.

Procedure

Experiment #3: Selection and Formulation

Use the 8 oz. color bottle and mix 1 oz. of 40 volume hydrogen peroxide with 1 oz. distilled water.

1. Use the 100 volume hydrogen peroxide chart to find the appropriate results.

2. Label and document results on the Experiment Results Sheet at the end of the chapter.

Procedure

Experiment #4: Selection and Formulation

Use the 8 oz. color bottle and mix 1 ½ oz. of 100 volume hydrogen peroxide and 2 ½ oz. of distilled water.

1. Use the 100 volume hydrogen peroxide chart to find the appropriate results.

2. Label and document results on the Experiment Results Sheet at the end of the chapter.

3. Answer the end-of-chapter Review Questions for this experiment.

Experiment Results Sheet and Review Questions

Varying Volumes of Hydrogen Peroxide

Experiment Results Sheet

Experiment 1 _____   Experiment 2 _____

H_2O_2 Used *: _____ H_2O_2 Used *: _____

Water Added: _____   Water Added: _____

Result: _____   Result: _____

_____   _____

Experiment 3 _____   Experiment 4 _____

H_2O_2 Used *: _____ H_2O_2 Used *: _____

Water Added: _____   Water Added: _____

Result: _____   Result: _____

_____   _____

* Label hydrogen peroxide (H_2O_2) used according to both quantity and volume.

Experiment Results Sheet and Review Questions

Varying Volumes of Hydrogen Peroxide

Review Questions

1. What does volume refer to?

2. How do you determine the lifting or depositing capabilities of H_2O_2 when it is mixed with color?

3. How do you determine the end volume of uneven or odd numbered peroxide volumes when they are mixed with color?

4. Why would you dilute peroxide with water?

5. What volumes of peroxide provide medium lift? High lift?

4 Hair Color Analysis

Learning Objectives

After completing this chapter, you should be able to:

- solve common hair-color-correction problems.
- explain the role and importance of the strand test.
- compensate for porosity problems when creating formulations.
- demonstrate how to neutralize the effects of chlorine.
- calculate the proper timing for color formulations.
- explain how to blend gray.

This chapter is designed to help you analyze the many color corrective situations you will face each day. It will explore some of the most common situations that arise during coloring services and their possible solutions. No single solution is always correct because so many variables come into play whenever human hair is involved.

At this point, you have learned what the level system is and how to use it, the difference between a shade of color and a level of color, and how to use hydrogen peroxide to ensure your coloring success. But, without the ability to analyze the head of hair you are working on, your success will be limited because many factors can change your choice of possible solutions. As you progress through the problems in this chapter, you'll learn to identify and address those factors.

Problem Solving

Problem #1

The client is a natural level 5 ash tone.

The ends are oxidized to a level 7 orange.

The hair has been permed repeatedly.

This client has virgin hair, where color is concerned.

The client does not like the orange ends.

Possible Solutions:

Answer 1

Apply blue-base level 5 semi-permanent color to the oxidized ends only and process according to the manufacturer's directions.

Caution: Do a strand test, using a small amount of color on a section of the ends to determine the timing needed for best results. Also, depending on the product you use and its pigment content, you may need to use a product that is one level darker or lighter, depending on the end's porosity.

Answer 2

Apply blue-base level 5 permanent color to the oxidized ends only. Now process according to instructions in Chapter 2. (See examples 1 and 2 and their explanations on pages 23–24, and Figs. 2.2 and 2.4 for a review of this subject.)

Caution: With this solution, you must consider the hair's porosity to achieve good color penetration. Again, do a strand test first. This will reveal any contributing factors you may have missed and will ensure the best results.

Answer 3

Add a plastic or vinyl polymer color to the neutralizer and apply to each rod during the client's next perm service.

Caution: If you choose this solution, remember that it is a temporary one. If the ends are in bad condition, the color could grab the base color. Artificial base color can overpower the natural pigment because it coats the cuticle. If this happens, the only way to remove it is by applying perm solution to the ends for three to five minutes and rinsing in warm water. You will need to reperm this client's hair if the above happens. Again, to be safe, do a strand test.

Problem #2

The client is a natural level 7 blond.

The client's ends are green.

The client's hair has been permed repeatedly.

The client has virgin hair where color is concerned.

The client swims all summer.

Answer 1

Apply a level 7 red, temporary color to the green areas. Process according to the manufacturer's directions.

Caution: Remember the cause of this problem is that the over-porous permed hair has grabbed chlorine. Do a strand test to be safe.

Answer 2

Apply a level 7 red permanent color to the green areas. Do a strand test first.

Caution: There is no guarantee that this answer will work; do a strand test first.

Answer 3

Apply at least three, 20-minute, depth protein conditioning treatments. Rinse in warm water after each treatment.

Caution: The hair's excessive porosity is the reason the chlorine attached to the ends. Do not use an oil-base conditioner, because it will coat the hair and compound the problem.

Problem #3

The client's hair is a natural level 6 ash brown.

The client's hair has level 6 red streaks.

The client's hair is not permed or colored.

The client shampoos, blows dry, and curls her hair everyday.

Answer 1

Apply a level 6 green temporary color to the red streaks. Process according to the manufacturer's directions.

Caution: Do a strand test to be safe.

Answer 2

Apply a level 6 green permanent color to the red streaks only.

Caution: Do a strand test to be safe.

Answer 3

Apply a green-base, plastic, semi-permanent color to red streaks. Process according to the manufacturer's directions.

Caution: Do a strand test first. Be prepared to remove this color with perm solution if results are unsatisfactory. Process three to five minutes and rinse with hot water.

Problem #4

The client's hair is a natural level 4.

The client's hair is 40 percent gray.

The client's hair is permed.

The client wishes to cover gray only.

Answer 1

Use a level 4 semi-permanent color. Apply to the entire head and process according to the manufacturer's directions.

Caution: Do a strand test first to be safe. Remember that color can grab onto gray hair or may only stain it.

Answer 2

Use a level 3 or 4 permanent color. Apply to entire head. Process according to the manufacturer's directions.

Caution: Do a strand test on the gray hair first to ensure proper results. If the gray hair is coarse, you may need to use 30 or 20 volume hydrogen peroxide to achieve proper penetration.

Answer 3

Use a level 4 permanent color. Use water or 5 volume hydrogen peroxide if hair is very porous from repeating perming.

Caution: Remember to do a strand test and use a neutral base color for best results.

Problem #5

The client's hair is a natural level 7 ash blond.

The client's hair is 20 percent gray, primarily around the face.

The client wishes to blend in the gray.

Answer 1

Use a level 7 neutral-base, semi-permanent color. Follow the manufacturer's directions.

Caution: Do a strand test on a small gray section and process accordingly.

Answer 2

Use a level 7 neutral-base permanent color. Remember that color can grab onto gray if the hair is overly porous.

Caution: Do a strand test on the gray hair to ensure proper penetration.

Answer 3

Use a level 6 neutral-base permanent color. Use a weave technique in gray areas only, to blend them into the natural hair color.

Caution: Do a strand test first to ensure proper results. Remember that the volume of hydrogen peroxide you use will depend on the porosity of the hair.

Any given problem can have many solutions. When in doubt, try your first solution with a strand test and record the results. If the results are not satisfactory, analyze why and try your next solution, recording those results. Continue in this manner until you reach the proper answer with the desired results. Then, and only then, proceed with a whole head application. This method may be time-consuming, but you will gain a satisfied client who will recommend you to her friends as a skilled colorist.

According to market research, each client is worth $1,500 a year to a stylist. If you lose a client, you also lose her friends and her co-workers, who rely on her recommendation. As you build your analytical skills, you build your future client base.

5 Corrective Color Solutions

Learning Objectives

After completing this chapter, you should be able to:

- analyze problem situation hair.
- suggest appropriate corrective solutions.
- explain the roles of texture and porosity in corrective color.
- define the type of hair that always has some degree of porosity.
- determine the effect of hair diameter on processing time.
- identify situations when adding conditioner to color is desirable.
- explain the major factors to consider when formulating color.

You will encounter varied and complex color situations in the salon. By putting her hair in your hands for coloring, a client commits the ultimate act of trust. To help you live up to that trust, this chapter explores a full spectrum of situations that take into account a cross section of problems. Look at the problems each situation poses one at a time, then solve them one at a time, in order of importance. The answers suggested in this chapter are by no means the only possible solutions in a given situation; they are only the most obvious possibilities.

Continued use of the theories explored in this chapter will allow you to become a more confident colorist and to develop analytical skills that will serve you throughout your career.

Salon coloring services generally fall into five basic categories. Regardless of the category, texture and porosity are always an important factor. Following are the categories and the textural and porosity variables associated with them.

Natural Hair:

fine texture — small diameter with little or no cuticle layer

medium texture — normal diameter with three or more cuticle layers

coarse texture — large diameter with many cuticle layers

---

very porous — hair will retain moisture and is difficult to dry

normal porosity — hair will retain some moisture but dries easily

no porosity — hair will not retain moisture and dries very quickly

Gray Hair:

fine texture — small diameter with little or no cuticle

normal texture — normal diameter and three or more cuticle layers

coarse texture — large diameter with many cuticle layers; difficult to perm

---

very porous — hair will retain moisture and is very difficult to dry normal porosity — hair will retain some moisture but dries easily

no porosity — hair will not retain moisture and dries very quickly

Permed Hair:

fine texture — small diameter with little or no cuticle

normal texture — normal diameter with three or more cuticle layers

coarse texture — large diameter with many cuticle layers

---

very porous — hair will retain moisture and is difficult to dry

normal porosity — hair will retain some moisture but dries easily

no porosity — hair will not retain moisture and dries very quickly

Colored Hair:

fine texture — small diameter with little or no cuticle

normal texture — normal diameter with three or more cuticle layers

coarse texture — large diameter with many cuticle layers; difficult to color

---

very porous — hair will retain moisture and is very difficult to dry

normal porosity — hair will retain some moisture but dries easily no porosity — hair will not retain moisture and dries very quickly; highly unusual in this category

Bleached Hair:

fine texture — small diameter with little or no cuticle

normal texture — normal diameter with three or more cuticle layers

coarse texture — large diameter with many cuticle layers

---

very porous — hair will retain moisture and is very difficult; normal in this category

normal porosity — hair will retain some moisture and dries easily; unusual in this category

no porosity — all bleached hair has some degree of porosity

Use the preceding general categories to identify your client's hair texture, porosity, and general condition before you perform any coloring services. The following examples are true-to-life situations that demonstrate the roles of porosity and texture in narrowing the color decision.

Examples

Example 1

The client is a natural level 5 (ash tone).

The client's ends are oxidized to a level 7 (orange).

The client's hair has been permed repeatedly.

The client has virgin hair where color is concerned.

The client does not like the orange ends.

The client's texture is fine.

The client's hair is very porous.

The client's hair is in poor condition.

An analysis of all the color factors leads to the decision that pre- and post-color conditioning treatments are a must. You also may want to add a maximum of 1/2 oz. animal protein conditioner to your coloring formula. This allows you to condition the hair while you are coloring it.

Caution: Do not use an oil-base or polymer conditioner. These conditioners will inhibit the color molecules, and they will not penetrate properly.

Example 2

The client's hair is a natural level 4.

The client's hair is 40 percent gray.

The client's hair is permed.

The client wishes to cover the gray only.

The client's texture is coarse.

The client's hair is normally porous.

The client's hair is in dry to normal condition.

These extra factors lead to the decision that 30 or 40 volume hydrogen peroxide will work best. (See Chapter 4, Problem 4, Answer 2 for more information.) 30 or 40 volume hydrogen peroxide is the correct choice because the hair has a coarse texture and the diameter is large, indicating that it will take longer for the color to oxidize or penetrate through the thick cuticle layer.

Example 3

The client's hair is a natural level 7 (ash blond).

The client's hair is 20 percent gray, primarily around the face.

The client wishes to blend the gray.

The client's hair is permed.

The client's texture is normal.

The client's hair is very porous.

The client's hair is in poor condition.

See Chapter 4, Problem 5, for possible solutions. If you selected Answer 3, remember that the volume of hydrogen peroxide you will need is 5 or 10. The use of animal protein conditioner in the color formula is optional; conditioning can be performed after the coloring service.

Example 4

The client's hair is a natural level 4.

The client's hair is 60 percent gray.

The client's hair is relaxed (ebony hair).

The client wishes to blend the gray and achieve a level 6, warm tone.

The client's texture is normal.

The client's porosity is normal.

The client's hair is in dry to normal condition.

The client has 1 ½ inch of new growth.

This represents one of the more unusual situations you will encounter. The following are recommendations; you may find other solutions that work equally well. First, relax the new growth with a normal strength relaxer. Next, condition with a moisturizing conditioner for at least 20 minutes. Then apply a level 8 blue-base color. You might need to add extra color pigment to ensure proper deposit. Use 20 or 30 volume hydrogen peroxide for ample oxidation time. In this instance, regular conditioning treatments are important.

A blue-base color is the correct choice, because at level 6 the remaining pigment contribution is red-orange. The client wishes to be a warm level 6, so a blue-base color will neutralize the orange at level 6, leaving a cool red, which is a softer tone.

Example 5

The client's hair is a natural level 5 (red).

The client's hair is permed.

The client wishes to be a level 5 (ash).

The client's texture is normal.

The client's hair is very porous.

The client's hair is dry and in very poor condition.

Since the client desires an ash tone, a green-base color will neutralize the undesirable red. The correct level is 5, and, because the hair has been chemically processed, 5 volume hydrogen peroxide is indicated. An animal protein conditioner added to the color mixture is also indicated. Mixing conditioner with the color will help it penetrate the cortex of the hair, strengthening it. Once oxidation is complete and the color is shampooed out, the hair will be in better condition than it was. This improvement in the internal structure of the hair shaft will help prevent fading. A good moisturizer used at home between salon visits and a pH-balanced shampoo of 4.5 to 5.5 will maintain the newly improved condition.

As you analyze all the factors that affect a color decision, remember that in some circumstances no color service is the best decision. If hair is in very poor condition, a "chemical vacation" with regular conditioning treatments will restore hair until another strand test can be performed — usually in a month or two.

6 Lighteners and Bleach

Learning Objectives

After completing this chapter, you should be able to:

- explain when to use bleach or lightener.
- describe the characteristics of gel lighteners.
- name the disadvantages of cream lighteners.
- account for the pH levels of different types of lighteners.
- define when oil lighteners should and should not be used.
- describe the advantages and disadvantages of powder lighteners.
- plan a course of action for any corrective color situation.
- explain why levels 11 and 12 are not true color levels.
- determine the correct timing for any type of lightener.

Double process blonding is the only way to achieve certain shades of blond on clients whose hair is naturally dark. While hair color advancements have created high lift products, reducing the need for bleaching, a small percentage of clients still require or opt for bleaching and then having a toner applied — a two step process.

Bleach is more commonly used today in frosting, weaving, foiling, or highlighting in a single process. This was not the case in decades past; in fact, the opposite was true. While the demand for bleaching lessens each year, as technical advances in hair color are made, understanding lighteners and bleach is still important. They are useful tools that can be used to achieve a variety of effects, particularly when highlighting — and knowledge of bleaches rounds out your color chemical knowledge.

Gel Lighteners

Gel lighteners most often come in a tube and have a lower pH than most lighteners. They are best used for on-the-scalp lightening or for foiling and weaving techniques. Gel lighteners do not lift as quickly as cream or oil lighteners do, and because they have a lower pH, they are not recommended for inclusion in color formulas.

Gel lighteners also have certain disadvantages. You must use a booster with them, and their lower pH causes them to react or lift more slowly. When using gel mixtures on the scalp, do not use peroxide volumes above 30.

Oil Lighteners

Oil lighteners are normally for use when lightening on the scalp. They are clear or blue, and are packaged in plastic or glass bottles. Their advantage is their steady lifting or lightening action. They can also be mixed into your color formula in small amounts for extra lifting.

Some of their disadvantages are that you have to add a booster to increase their pH level if you choose to use them instead of color, and they will do more damage to the internal structure of the hair shaft than color will. When using oil lighteners on the scalp, never use hydrogen peroxide volumes above 30.

Cream Lighteners

Cream lighteners are very similar to oil lighteners. They are usually cloudy, range in color from blue to violet to green, and are always packaged in plastic or glass bottles. One of the advantages of cream lighteners is that they have steady lifting or lightening power.

Disadvantages are that they require a booster to increase their level, and if you choose to use cream lighteners instead of color, they will affect the internal structure of the hair shaft more harshly. When using them on the scalp, never use hydrogen peroxide volumes above 30.

Powder Lighteners

Powder lighteners usually come in a can, but can come in packets or plastic bags. The advantage of using them is that they have a pH of 10.2 or more, permitting excellent lift in less time than color requires. They are normally mixed with 20 volume hydrogen peroxide.

One disadvantage of powder lighteners is that they have a tendency to swell or "creep," bleeding onto hair not intended to be bleached. They are used for lightening off the scalp only.

The following examples illustrate situations frequently seen in the salon. They will help you learn to analyze each of your color clients' hair and plan a course of action before you apply the color formula to hair. It is easier to solve problems before the actual application; this is a learned habit. With practice it will become second nature to you. Remember, if you are uncertain about any of the color solutions offered in this book, go back and re-read the applicable material. If you are skeptical, test the theories on samples of hair that you have obtained from clients. Risk-free experimentation is one of the best ways to learn.

Before you move on to the experiments at the end of this chapter, examine the following chart. In this remaining pigment chart, two new levels are included — levels 11 and 12. They are actually forms of lighteners and do not represent a color level. Manufacturers may refer to them as color, but since they have more than 90 percent lifting capabilities and considerably less than 10 percent depositing capabilities, they are considered lighteners and bleaches, for chemical purposes. These "color" lighteners, if you will, are similar to gel lighteners but do not require boosters for lightening or lifting. They also have a higher pH than color levels 1–10. If there are any terms you do not understand, please refer to the glossary of terms at the end of this chapter. Continue expanding your knowledge of coloring, and accomplished corrective coloring will become an enjoyable, rewarding specialty. There is no problem that cannot be solved by the advanced, professional, hair colorist.

Level System Including Color Lighteners

Remaining Pigment Chart

Level 1 Blue

Dark Brown= _____Blue Browns

Level 2 Blue Violet

Level 3 Violet

Level 4 Red Violet

Medium Brown= _____Red Browns

Level 5 Red

Level 6 Red Orange

Dark Blond= _____ Red Blonds

Level 7 Orange

Level 8 Yellow Orange

Light Blond= _____Yellow Blond

Level 9 Yellow

Level 10 Pale Yellow

Lightest Blond= _____Pale Yellow Blond

Level 11 Palest Yellow

White = _____White

Level 12

Experiment Instruction Sheets
Lightening Comparisons

Objective — Experiment #1

To determine the amount of time needed to lighten swatches to the white stage using gel lighteners.

Hair Swatches Needed

2 hair swatches of the following levels:

- Level 3 — Brown
- Level 7 — Blond

Labeling Hair Swatches

Label each swatch to indicate its natural color.

Materials Needed

- Gel lightener
- 20 volume H_2O_2
- One standard mixing bowl
- One standard timer

Selection Formulation

1. Select the level 7 swatch.
2. Mix gel lightener with 20 volume hydrogen peroxide in the mixing bowl, following the manufacturer's directions.

Procedure

1. Immerse the level 7 blond swatch in the gel lightener and begin timing until the swatch is white.

2. Mount swatch on the Experiment Results Sheet at the end of the chapter, and document the timing.

3. Repeat formulation and procedure, using the level 3 swatch.

Objective — Experiment #2

To determine the time needed to lighten level 3 to level 7 using cream lightener.

Hair Swatches Needed

2 hair swatches of the following levels:

- Level 3 — Brown
- Level 7 — Blond

Labeling Hair Swatches

Label each swatch to indicate its natural color.

Materials Needed

- Cream lightener
- 20 volume H_2O_2
- One standard mixing bowl
- One standard timer

Selection and Formulation

1. Select the level 3 swatch.
2. Mix cream lightener with 20 volume hydrogen peroxide, following the manufacturer's directions.

Procedure

1. Immerse level 3 brown swatch into the cream lightener and begin timing until level 7 blond is reached.

2. Mount the swatch on the Experiment Results Sheet at the end of the chapter and document the timing.

Objective — Experiment #3

To determine the time needed to lighten swatches to the white stage, using cream lighteners.

Hair Swatches Needed

- Level 3 — Brown
- Level 7 — Blond

Labeling Hair Swatches

Label each swatch with its natural color.

Materials Needed

- Cream lightener
- 20 volume H_2O_2
- One standard mixing bowl
- One standard timer

Selection and Formulation

1. Select the level 7 swatch.
2. Mix cream lightener with 20 volume hydrogen peroxide, in the mixing bowl, following the manufacturer's directions.

Procedure

1. Immerse level 7 blond swatch into the cream lightener and begin timing until the swatch is white.

2. Mount swatch on the Experiment Results Sheet at the end of the chapter and document the timing.

3. Repeat formulation and procedure, using the level 3 swatch.

Objective — Experiment #4

Determine the time needed to lighten level 3 to level 7 using oil lightener.

Hair Swatches Needed

2 hair swatches of the following levels:

- Level 3 — Brown
- Level 7 — Blond

Labeling Hair Swatches

Label each swatch to indicate its natural color.

Materials Needed

- Oil lightener
- 20 volume H_2O_2
- One standard mixing bowl
- One standard timer

Selection and Formulation

1. Select the level 3 swatch.

2. Mix oil lightener with 20 volume hydrogen peroxide in the mixing bowl, following the manufacturer's directions.

Procedure

1. Immerse the level 3 brown swatch into the oil lightener and begin timing until level 7 blond is reached.

2. Mount the swatch on the Experiment Results Sheet at the end of the chapter and document the timing.

Objective — Experiment #5

To determine the amount of time needed to lighten swatches to the white stage, using oil lightener.

Hair Swatches Needed

2 hair swatches of the following levels:

- Level 3 — Brown
- Level 7 — Blond

Labeling Hair Swatches

Label each swatch to indicate its natural color.

Materials Needed

- Oil lightener
- 20 volume H_2O_2
- One standard mixing bowl
- One standard timer

Selection and Formulation

1. Select the level 7 swatch.
2. Mix oil lightener and 20 volume hydrogen peroxide in the mixing bowl, following the manufacturer's directions.

Procedure

1. Immerse the level 7 blond swatch into the oil lightener and begin timing until the swatch is white.

2. Mount the swatch on the Experiment Results Sheet at the end of the chapter and document the timing.

3. Repeat formulation and procedure, using the level 3 swatch.

Objective — Experiment 6

To determine the time needed to lighten level 3 to level 7, using powder lightener.

Hair Swatches Needed

2 hair swatches of the following levels:

- Level 3 — Brown
- Level 7 — Blond

Labeling Hair Swatches

Label each swatch to indicate its natural color.

Materials Needed

- Powder lightener
- 20 volume H_2O_2
- One standard mixing bowl
- One standard timer

Selection and Formulation

1. Select the level 3 swatch.
2. Mix powder lightener with 20 volume hydrogen peroxide in the mixing bowl, following the manufacturer's directions.

Procedure

1. Immerse the level 3 brown swatch into the powder lightener and begin timing until level 7 blond is reached.

2. Mount the swatch on the Experiment Results Sheet at the end of the chapter and document the timing.

Objective — Experiment #7

To determine the amount of time needed to lighten swatches to the white stage, using powder lighteners.

Hair Swatches Needed

- Level 3 — Brown
- Level 7 — Blond

Labeling Hair Swatches

Label each swatch to indicate its natural color.

Materials Needed

- Powder lightener
- 20 volume H_2O_2
- One standard mixing bowl
- One standard timer

Selection and Formulation

1. Select the level 7 swatch.

2. Mix powder lightener with 20 volume hydrogen peroxide in mixing bowl, following the manufacturer's directions.

Procedure

1. Immerse the level 7 hair swatch into the powder lightener and begin timing until the swatch is white.

2. Mount swatch on the Experiment Results Sheet at the end of the chapter and document the timing.

3. Repeat the formulation and procedure, using the level 3 swatch.

4. Answer end-of-chapter Review Questions for this experiment.

Experiment Results Sheets and Review Questions

Lightening Comparisons

Experiment Results Sheet — Odd-Numbered Experiments

Experiment 1
Gel Lightener

Level 7   Level 3

Experiment 3
Cream Lightener

Level 7   Level 3

time: time:

time: time:

Experiment 5
Oil Lightener

Level 7   Level 3

Experiment 7
Powder Lightener

Level 7   Level 3

time: time:

time: time:

Slowest time lightening level 7 to white:

_____

Slowest time lightening level 3 to white:

_____

Fastest time lightening level 7 to white:

_____

Fastest time lightening level 3 to white:

_____

Significant differences in lightening levels:

_____

_____

_____

Comments:_____

_____

_____

Experiment Results Sheets and Review Questions

Lightening Comparisons

Experiment Results Sheet — Even-Numbered Experiments

Experiment 2	*Experiment 4*	*Experiment 6*
Cream Lightener	Oil Lightener	Powder Lightener

time: time: time:

Fastest achieving level 7: _____

Slowest achieving level 7: _____

Closest visually to level 7 sample: _____

Comments:_____

_____

_____

Experiment Results Sheets and Review Questions

Lightening Comparisons

___

Review Questions

1. Name the types of lighteners and their advantages. Disadvantages?

2. How does level affect the timing it takes to achieve white?

3. How does the lightener used affect the ability to lighten from level 3 to level 7?

4. Give three examples of how lighteners are used in hair coloring.

5. What are levels 11 and 12?

Glossary

We include this glossary with the intention of helping to standardize the language for hair color. It has been prepared and authorized by the International Haircolor Exchange, an organization interested in furthering hair color education.

accelerator: (See activator.)

accent color: A concentrated color product that can be added to permanent, semi-permanent, or temporary hair color to intensify or tone down the color. Another word for concentrate.

acid: An aqueous (water based) solution having a pH less than 7.0 on the pH scale.

activator: An additive used to quicken the action or progress of a chemical. Another word for booster, accelerator, protinator, or catalyst.

alkaline: An aqueous (water based) solution having a pH greater than 7.0 on the pH scale. The opposite of acid.

allergy: A reaction due to extreme sensitivity to certain foods or chemicals.

allergy test: A test to determine the possibility or degree of sensitivity, also known as a patch test, predisposition test, or skin test.

amino acids: The group of molecules that the body uses to synthesize protein. There are 22 different amino acids found in living protein that serve as units of structure.

ammonia: A colorless, pungent gas composed of hydrogen and nitrogen; in water solution it is called ammonia water. Used in hair color to swell the cuticle. When mixed with hydrogen peroxide, activates the oxidation process on melanin and allows the melanin to decolorize.

ammonium hydroxide: An alkaline solution of ammonia in water, commonly used in the manufacture of permanent hair color, lightener preparations, and hair relaxers.

analysis (hair): An examination of the hair to determine its condition and natural color. (See consultation; condition.)

aqueous: Descriptive term for water solution or any medium that is largely composed of water.

ash: A tone or shade dominated by greens, blues, violets, or grays. May be used to counteract unwanted warm tones.

base (alkali): (See pH; alkaline.)

base color: (See color base.)

bleeding: Seepage of tint/lightener from foil or cap due to improper application.

blending: A merging of one tint or tone with another.

blonding: A term applied to lightening the hair.

bonds: The means by which atoms are joined together to make molecules.

booster: (See activator.)

brassy tone: Red, orange, or gold tones in the hair.

breakage: A condition when hair splits and breaks off.

build-up: Repeated coatings on the hair shaft.

catalyst: A substance used to alter the speed of a chemical reaction.

caustic: Strongly alkaline materials. At very high pH levels, can burn or destroy protein or tissue by chemical action.

certified color: A color that meets certain standards for purity and is certified by the FDA.

cetyl alcohol: Fatty alcohol used as an emollient. It is also used as a stabilizer for emulsion systems and in hair color and cream developer as a thickener.

chelating stabilizer: A molecule that binds metal ions and renders them inactive.

chemical change: Alteration in the chemical composition of a substance.

citric acid: Organic acid derived from citrus fruits and used for pH adjustment. Primarily used to adjust the acid-alkaline balance. Has some antioxidant and preservative qualities. Used medicinally as a mild astringent.

coating: Residue left on the outside of the hair shaft.

color: Visual sensation caused by light.

color additive: (See accent color.)

color base: The combination of dyes making up the tonal foundation of a specific hair color.

color life: The amount of change natural or artificial pigment undergoes when lightened by a substance.

color mixing: Combining two or more shades together for a custom color.

color refresher: 1. Color applied to midshaft and ends to give a more uniform color appearance to the hair. 2. Color applied by a shampoo-in method to enhance the natural color. Also called color wash, color enhancer.

color remover: A product designed to remove artificial pigment from the hair.

color test: The process of removing product from a hair strand to monitor the progress of color development during tinting or lightening.

color wheel: The arrangement of primary, secondary, and tertiary colors in the order of their relationships to each other. A tool for formulating.

complementary colors: Primary and secondary colors positioned opposite each other on the color wheel. When these two colors are combined, they create a neutral color. Combinations are as follows: blue/orange, red/green, yellow/violet.

concentrate: (See accent color.)

condition: The existing state of the hair; elasticity, strength, texture, porosity, and evidence of previous treatments.

consultation: Verbal communication with a client to determine desired result. (See analysis, hair.)

contributing pigment: The current level and tone of the hair. Refers to both natural contributing pigment and decolorized (or lightened) contributing pigment. (See undertone.)

cool tones: (See ash.)

corrective coloring: The process of correcting an undesirable color.

cortex: The second layer of hair. A fibrous protein core of the hair fiber, containing melanin pigment.

coverage: Reference to the ability of a color product to color gray, white, or other colors of hair.

cuticle: The translucent protein outer layer of the hair fiber.

cysteic acid: A chemical substance in the hair fiber, produced by the interaction of hydrogen peroxide with the disulfide bond (cystine).

cystine: The disulfide amino acid that joins protein chains together.

D & C colors: Colors selected from a certified list approved by the Food and Drug Administration for use in drug and cosmetic products.

decolorize: A chemical process involving the lightening of the natural color pigment or artificial color from the hair.

degree: Term used to describe various units of measurement.

dense: Thick, compact, or crowded.

deposit: Describes the color product in terms of its ability to add color pigment to the hair. Color added equals deposit.

deposit-only color: A category of color products between permanent and semi-permanent colors. Formulated only to deposit color, not lift. These products contain oxidation dyes and utilize low volume developer.

depth: The lightness or darkness of a specific hair color. (See value; level.)

developer: An oxidizing agent, usually hydrogen peroxide, which reacts chemically with coloring material to develop color molecules and create a change in natural hair color.

development tine (oxidation period): The time required for a permanent color or lightener to completely develop.

diffused: Broken down, scattered; not limited to one spot.

direct dye: A pre-formed color that dyes the fiber directly without the need for oxidation.

discoloration: The development of undesired shades through chemical reaction.

double process: A technique requiring two separate procedures during which the hair is decolorized or pre-lightened with a lightener before the depositing color is applied.

drab: Term used to describe hair color shades containing no red or gold. (See ash; dull.)

drabber: Concentrated color, used to reduce red or gold highlights.

dull: A word used to describe hair or hair color without sheen.

dye: Artificial pigment.

dye intermediate: A material that develops into color only after reaction with a developer (hydrogen peroxide). Also known as oxidation dyes.

dye solvents or dye remover: (See color remover.)

dye stock: (See color base.)

elasticity: The ability of the hair to stretch and return to normal.

enzyme: A protein molecule found in living cells that initiates a chemical process.

fade: To lose color through exposure to the elements or other factors.

fillers: 1. A color product used as a color refresher or to fill damaged hair in preparation for hair coloring. 2. Any liquid-like substance to help fill a void. (See color refresher.)

formulas: Mixtures of two or more ingredients.

formulate: The art of mixing to create a blend or balance of two or more ingredients.

gray hair: Hair with decreasing amounts of natural pigment. Hair with no natural pigment is actually white. White hairs look gray when mingled with pigmented hair.

hair: A slender, threadlike outgrowth of the skin of the head and body.

hair root: That part of the hair contained within the follicle, below the surface of the scalp.

hair shaft: Visible part of each strand of hair. It is made up of an outer layer called the cuticle, an innermost layer called medulla, and an in-between layer called the cortex. The cortex layer is where color changes are made.

hard water: Water that contains minerals and metallic salts as impurities.

henna: A plant-extracted coloring that produces bright shades of red. The active ingredient is lawsone. Henna permanently colors the hair by coating and penetrating the hair shaft. (See progressive dye.)

high lift tinting: A single-process color with a higher degree of lightening action and a minimal amount of color deposit.

highlighting: The introduction of a lighter color in small, selected sections to increase lightness of hair. Generally not strongly contrasting from the natural color.

hydrogen peroxide: An oxidizing chemical made up of 2 parts hydrogen and 2 parts oxygen (H_2O_2) used to aid the processing of permanent hair color and lighteners. Also referred to as a developer; available in liquid or cream.

level: A unit of measurement used to evaluate the lightness or darkness of a color, excluding tone.

level system: In haircoloring, a system colorists use to analyze the lightness or darkness of a hair color.

lift: The lightening action of a hair color or lightening product on the hair's natural pigment.

lightener: The chemical compound that lightens the hair by dispersing, dissolving, and decolorizing the natural hair pigment. (See pre-lighten.)

lightening: (See decolorize.)

line of demarcation: An obvious difference between two colors on the hair shaft.

litmus paper: A chemically treated paper used to test the acidity or alkalinity of products.

medulla: The center structure of the hair shaft. Little is known about its actual function.

melanin: The tiny grains of pigment in the hair cortex that create natural hair color.

melanocytes: Cells in the hair bulb that manufacture melanin.

melanoprotein: The protein coating of a melanosome.

melanosome: Protein-coated granule containing melanin.

metallic dyes: Soluble metal salts such as lead, silver, and bismuth that produce colors on the hair fiber by progressive build-up and exposure to air.

modifier: A chemical found as an ingredient in permanent hair colors. Its function is to alter the dye intermediates.

molecule: Two or more atoms chemically joined together; the smallest part of a compound.

neutral: 1. A color balanced between warm and cool, which does not reflect a highlight of any primary or secondary color. 2. Also refers to a pH of 7.

neutralization: The process that counterbalances or cancels the action of an agent or color.

neutralize: Render neutral; counterbalance of action or influence. (See neutral.)

new growth: The part of the hair shaft that is between previously chemically treated hair and the scalp.

nonalkaline: (See acid.)

off-the-scalp lightener: Generally a stronger lightener, usually in powder form, not to be used directly on the scalp.

on-the-scalp lightener: A liquid, cream, or gel form of lightener that can be used directly on the scalp.

opaque: Allowing no light to shine through.

outgrowth: (See new growth.)

overlap: Occurs when the application of color or lightener goes beyond the line of demarcation.

over-porosity: The condition where hair reaches an undesirable stage of porosity, requiring correction.

oxidation: 1. The reaction of dye intermediates found in hair coloring developers with hydrogen peroxide. 2. The interaction of hydrogen peroxide on the natural pigment.

oxidative hair color: A product containing oxidation dyes that require hydrogen peroxide to develop the permanent color.

para-tint: A tint made from oxidation dyes.

para-phenylenediamine: An oxidation dye used in most permanent hair colors, often abbreviated as P.P.D.

patch test: A test required by the Food and Drug Act. Made by applying a small amount of the hair coloring preparation to the skin of the arm or behind the ear to determine possible allergies (hypersensitivity). Also called predisposition or skin test.

penetrating color: Color that enters or penetrates the cortex or second layer of the hair shaft.

permanent color: 1. Hair color products that do not wash out by shampooing. 2. A category of hair color products mixed with developer that create a lasting color change.

peroxide: (See hydrogen peroxide.)

peroxide residue: Traces of peroxide left in the hair after treatment with lightener or tint.

persulfate: In hair coloring, a chemical ingredient commonly used in activators. It increases the speed of the decolorization process. (See activator.)

pH: The quality that expresses the acid/alkaline balance. A pH of 7 is the neutral value for pure water. Any pH below 7 is acidic; any pH above 7 is alkaline. The skin is mildly acidic and generally in the pH range of 4.5 to 5.5.

pH scale: A numerical scale from 0 (very acid) to 14 (very alkaline), used to describe the degree of acidity or alkalinity.

pigment: Any substance or matter used as coloring: natural or artificial hair color.

porosity: Ability of the hair to absorb water or other liquids.

powder lightener: (See off-the-scalp lightener.)

pre-bleaching: (See pre-lighten.)

predisposition test: (See patch test.)

pre-lighten: Generally the first step of double-process hair coloring. To lift or lighten the natural pigment. (See decolorize.)

pre-soften: The process of treating gray or very resistant hair to allow for better penetration of color.

primary colors: Pigments or colors that are fundamental and cannot be made by mixing colors together. Red, yellow, and blue are the primary colors.

prism: A transparent glass or crystal solid that breaks up white light into its component colors, the spectrum.

processing time: The time required for the chemical treatment to react on the hair.

progressive dyes or progressive dye system: 1. A coloring system that produces increased absorption with each application. 2. Color products that deepen or increase absorption over a period of time during processing.

regrowth: (See new growth.)

resistant hair: Hair that is difficult to penetrate with moisture or chemical solutions.

retouch: Application of color or lightening mixture to new growth of hair.

salt and pepper: The descriptive term for a mixture of dark and gray or white hair.

secondary color: Colors made by combining two primary colors in equal proportion: green, orange and violet are secondary colors.

semi-permanent hair coloring: Hair coloring that lasts through several shampoos. It penetrates the hair shaft and stains the cuticle layer, slowly diffusing out with each shampoo.

sensitivity: A skin highly reactive to the presence of a specific chemical. Skin reddens or becomes irritated shortly after application of the chemical. On removal of the chemical, the reaction subsides.

shade: 1. A term used to describe a specific color. 2. The visible difference between two colors.

sheen: The ability of the hair to shine, gleam, or reflect light.

single process color: Refers to an oxidative tint solution that lifts or lightens while also depositing color in one application. (See oxidative hair color.)

softening agent: A mild alkaline product applied prior to the color treatment, to increase porosity, swell the cuticle layer of the hair, and increase color absorption. Tint that has not been mixed with developer is frequently used. (See pre-soften.)

solution: A blended mixture of solid, liquid, or gaseous substances in a liquid medium.

solvent: Carrier liquid in which other components may be dissolved.

specialist: One who concentrates on one part, branch, or subject; or a professional.

spectrum: The series of colored bands diffracted and arranged in the order of their wavelengths by the passage of white light through a prism. Shading continuously from red (produced by the longest wave visible) to violet (produced by the shortest): Red, orange, yellow, green, blue, indigo and violet.

spot lightening: Color correcting using a lightening mixture to lighten darker areas.

stabilizer: General name for ingredient that prolongs lifetime, appearance, and performance of a product.

stage: A term used to describe a visible color change that natural hair goes through while being lightened.

stain remover: Chemical used to remove tint stains from skin.

strand test: Test given before treatment to determine development time, color result, and the ability of the hair to withstand the effects of chemicals.

stripping: (See color remover.)

surfactant: A short way of staying Surface Active Agent. A molecule that is composed of an oil-loving (oleophilic) part and a water-loving (hydrophilic) part. They act as a bridge to allow oil and water to mix. Wetting agents, emulsifiers, cleansers, solubilizers, dispersing aids, and thickeners are usually surfactants.

tablespoon: ½ of an ounce. 3 teaspoons.

teaspoon: ⅙ of an ounce. ⅓ of a tablespoon.

temporary coloring or temporary rinses: Color made from pre-formed dyes that are applied to the hair, but are readily removed with shampoo.

terminology: The special words or terms used in a specific science, art, or business.

tertiary colors: The mixture of a primary and an adjacent secondary color on the color wheel. Red-orange, yellow-orange, yellow-green, blue-green, blue-violet, red-violet. Also referred to as intermediary colors.

texture, hair: The diameter of an individual hair strand. Termed: coarse, medium or fine.

tint: Permanent oxidizing hair color product having the ability to lift and deposit color in the same process.

tint back: To return hair back to its original or natural color.

tone: A term used to describe the warmth or coolness in color.

toner: A pastel color to be used after pre-lightening.

toning: Adding color to modify the end result.

touch-up: (See retouch.)

translucent: The property of letting diffused light pass through.

tyrosine: The amino acid (tyrosine) that reacts together with the enzyme (tyrosinase) to form the hair's natural melanin.

tyrosinase: The enzyme (tyrosinase) that reacts together with the amino acid (tyrosine) to form the hair's natural melanin.

undertone: The underlying color that emerges during the lifting process of melanin that contributes to the end result. When lightening hair, a residual warmth in tone always occurs.

urea peroxide: A peroxide compound occasionally used in hair color. When added to an alkaline color mixture, it releases oxygen.

value: (See level; depth.)

vegetable color: A color derived from plant sources.

virgin hair: Natural hair that has not undergone any chemical or physical abuse.

viscosity: A term referring to the thickness of the solution.

volume: The concentration of hydrogen peroxide in water solution. Expressed as volumes of oxygen liberated per volume of solution. 20 volume peroxide would thus liberate 20 pints of oxygen gas for each pint of solution.

warm: Containing red, orange, yellow, or gold tones.

Appendix — Answers to Review Questions

Chapter 1

Creating Secondary Colors

1. The three primary colors are red, yellow, and blue.

2. The primary colors are basic, or true, colors.

3. Secondary colors are orange, green, and violet. They are created by mixing any two primary colors in equal proportions.

4. If you add the opposite of any secondary color, you neutralize it, and it becomes neutral brown or neutral blond.

5. Blue, red, and yellow.

6. Colorists use opposite colors on the color wheel to neutralize hair color.

Creating Tertiary Colors

1. Blue green, red orange, yellow green.

2. Add red-orange to it.

3. Between any primary and secondary color.

4. The deeper the pigment in the hair shaft, the harder it is to remove.

5. At least one primary color and one secondary color; equal parts.

Chapter 2

Determining Natural Level of Virgin Hair

1. The level system is a method of categorizing hair color numerically in relation to depth of color and lifting capabilities. It is used by hair-color manufacturers to standardize hair colors and number the bottles/tubes.

2. The color that will be left in the hair during the lifting process.

3. Red and orange.

4. Most displays show color selections on white hair swatches.

5. Natural brunettes could be levels 1, 2, 3, 4, or 5.

6. Knowing what colors are present will help the colorist choose the correct base color to either neutralize or enhance the color.

Determining Level of Chemically Treated Hair

1. Shade is specific tonal quality; as many as four shades can be in each level.

2. Level 1, blue; level 2, blue-violet; level 3, violet; level 4, red-violet.

3. Melanin is pigment in the hair cortex that creates natural hair color.

4. Lift in any color is directly related to its ammonia content. Deposit is directly related to dye content in the color bottle or tube.

5. Oxidation occurs when hydrogen peroxide loses an oxygen molecule.

Chapter 3

Varying Volumes of Hydrogen Peroxide

1. Volume means "by weight."
2. Add the total quantity of product used, then divide that sum into the volume of hydrogen peroxide used. The result is the lift or depositing capabilities of the hydrogen peroxide.
3. Divide the number 4 into the volume of hydrogen peroxide used.
4. To show that H_2O and H_2O_2 when combined in equal amounts will change H_2O_2. Fox example, 10 volume is now 5 volume; 20 volume is now 10 volume; 30 volume is now 15 volume.
5. Medium lift formula: 7–11 volume; high lift formula: 12–18 volume.

Chapter 4

No questions.

Chapter 5

No questions.

Chapter 6

Lightening Comparisons

1. Gel lighteners: advantages — have a lower pH than most lighteners; disadvantages — must use a booster with them, and they lift slowly. Oil lighteners: advantages — steady lifting action; disadvantages — do more damage to internal structure of hair shaft than color will. Cream lighteners: advantages — steady lifting power; disadvantages — require a booster to increase their level. Powder lighteners: advantages — excellent lift in less time than color; disadvantages — tendency to swell, or "creep."
2. The darker the level you start with, the more time you need to achieve white.

3. Lighteners are of different strengths, and some can lighten through more levels than others. For instance, oil bleaches are only appropriate when one or two levels of color lift are desired. The lightener used will also affect the length of time it takes to lighten from level 3 to level 7.

4. Lighteners are used for frosting, weaving, foiling, highlighting, or lightening hair.

5. White.